My Journey
From Gallbladder Attack to Recovery Without Surgery

By Joanne Elvira

This book is dedicated to you.

CONTENTS

PREFACE

This book is a recollection and memoir of my own experience of a gallbladder attack, the steps I took, the choices I had to make and how I went against all odds and avoided surgery.

By doing so, my diet and lifestyle changed, miraculously saving my gallbladder and improving my overall health. This book is about my journey from a gallbladder attack to health and wellness.

This is not a book of advice. I am not a medical expert.

But I am sharing this book to let my readers know that they too can face situations where they may need to make difficult choices. At the time I was unwell, I couldn't find any literature from people who had experienced gallstones and other problems with their gallbladder.

I want to share my journey with you so that you can understand that you have options. That if you are willing to go on the longer journey, you can see the results that I too experienced.

If I was able to get through it, I'm sure that you can too. You have chosen this book for a reason. I hope the information in the pages of this book will help you discover your inner strength to enable you to achieve lifelong health and wellness.

Good luck on your journey,
Joanne

1 - THE WAKE UP CALL

On the 14th day of August 2019, I was suddenly woken up with a pain in my abdomen. It was 2am. My first reaction was to reach for the Gaviscon. It made no difference. I took painkillers to no avail. By 6am I was in real agony. The pain had spread to my back, making it feel like a knife stabbing in my back.

The thought of going to hospital and having to wait hours to be attended to in emergency turned me off ringing the ambulance. I waited until my local family clinic opened. How I managed to endure the pain for so long is beyond belief.

When I rang my clinic at 8am I could barely speak. I was told by the secretary to see my GP immediately. I'm very lucky the clinic is just five minutes from my home. I rushed out my front door almost unconscious. My GP rang me an ambulance and I was admitted into hospital. I had to wait, sitting in a wheelchair, for a bed to become available.

While I was waiting, I was very disorientated and very much in pain. A male nurse asked me if I wanted a warm blanket. I realised that I was shaking. I don't know if it was the cold August air, or my mind racing, knowing how tired and sore I was, and how much I needed help.

The nurse threw the warm blanket over me and it was the most comforting and loveliest feeling coming upon my body and mind.

I hugged that blanket with a feeling of content, like the warm feeling you get when you hug a loved one, or a great friend, and for a while I was lost in bliss.

My eyes followed everyone and everything going on around the emergency ward. I had never felt so fragile in my entire life. Knowing I was alone, with no loved ones by my side to take care of me, made me anxious and insecure.

I have never liked hospitals as my perception of hospitals is they are for the sick. Knowing I was in one made me realise my life depended on being there. I encountered the most gentle, loving, caring nurses that came to my aid and helped me relax. My faith was placed upon them. At the same time I thought that in order to help myself, I needed to be strong. Observing those nurses taking care of the sick, needy, and frail calmed me down to a degree. Before all the drama I had been slowly losing hope in humanity. But in this moment, I had my faith restored.

"I believe there are angels among us, sent down to us from above. They come to you and me in our darkest hours, to show us how to live, to teach us how to give, to guide us with a light of love" - Helen Keller.

I am now really convinced that there are angels among us and I had the privilege to witness these angels first hand, performing acts of love and care. It almost brought tears to my eyes. I was so consumed by their care that I was starting to see through eyes that once had been blinded. I had experienced so much despair and emotional pain, and had been in an insecure state of mind, due to the realities of life which I had been finding hard to endure.

I had been given morphine, but the pain had not eased. I felt more relaxed though, and the thought that I was being looked after was so comforting.

When I finally got a bed, I was treated for the pain with more morphine. It eased the pain.

After numerous hours in hospital, and numerous tests, including an ultrasound, I was by then still tender under my ribs.

I was told the doctor would see me and he would explain to me the cause of the pain. When he came to see me, he explained that an 11mm stone was found stuck in my bile duct and I had inflammation in the gallbladder.

The doctor suggested surgical removal of my gallbladder. He explained the procedure would be done by keyhole surgery, which would be straightforward and would leave no scars. He also told me that I could live a normal life without a gallbladder.

At the time I was told this news, fortunately the stone in my bile duct had passed. The suggestion put to me by the doctor shocked me though. I definitely was not prepared to give the doctor the answer he probably hoped to hear straight away. I was highly afraid of surgery. I always had been.

Remembering my father's point of view about going under the knife, he would say surgery was the beginning of life-long medical intervention. Having some knowledge about nutrition and health myself, and realising I had been living a care-free existence, I was now paying for this with my health. Hearing the doctor's opinion, and thinking whether such a drastic procedure was necessary, I questioned if there were perhaps other alternatives.

After thinking through all these things, I quickly made the decision and told the doctor, "I am going to try and change my diet and lifestyle". He responded "I'll make you a follow-up appointment to return next week. This will give you some time to think about the choices and maybe reconsider going ahead with the procedure".

I was happy that the doctor accepted my answer. I would not have to see him for another week, during which time I could think about my decision thoroughly.

As I was getting dressed to go home, a nurse told me that if the stone in my bile duct had not passed, I would not have had a choice but would have had my gallbladder taken out there and then.

I consider myself very lucky that I was able to walk out of the hospital, and have a week to seek alternatives which would enable me to keep my gallbladder. These included booking a dietitian, engaging in exercise, reducing stress, and having a positive frame of mind.

After coming home, I felt tender for a few days and almost considered having my gallbladder removed. My GP was encouraging me to go ahead and have it taken out, but instead I decided to improve my health and keep my gallbladder.

I immediately started researching the function of the gallbladder, and taking in every little detail religiously. By examining the test results I had been given, I started to improve my cholesterol and everything else malfunctioning inside me. Eating well, exercising and improving my lifestyle made a huge impact on my health in just a short time. Realising this, I was happy to do as I believed, as they say "the proof is in the pudding".

Therefore, at my follow-up appointment, one week later, I had no doubt or hesitation in my mind as to which path I was going to take. I was keeping my gallbladder and improving my overall health. To this day, I have no doubt that I made the right decision.

A couple of weeks after my hospital say, I found the most adorable companion, a Pomeranian dog that motivated me to exercise. After reading the dog's description on a website, I was hesitant whether I was going to get him, as I had been looking for a female dog instead. But as soon as I saw him, I knew I was bringing him home.

I named him Tigger. He was four months old and has been with me ever since. He has improved my life because he is so active and we enjoy our walks together to this day.

2 - THE CAUSES AND THE CONSEQUENCES

My journey into unwellness took me two years but this is different for everybody. Previous to this, I ate well and exercised. I had never been overweight in my entire life, so this journey to unwellness was very unlike me. It shows that feelings of loneliness, stress and being emotionally unwell can be huge triggers to major illnesses in our body and mind. Not just the gallbladder.

The week before I was admitted to hospital, I had been feeling awfully depressed due to the break-up of my relationship with my ex-partner.

After over a decade of romance and happily living together, just like the blink of an eye, it all concluded. I don't know who was to blame. The last two years before our relationship ended, it had become unbearably complex. Complex to a degree that for our sanity and our peace of mind it was better and sensible to go our separate ways.

Having him move out left me a complete wreck. A void that consumed me immensely on a daily basis. A loneliness I could not bare.

Moving with the flow of life with no emotion, no desire, no interests.

Living in a state of unconsciousness, with a broken heart and a yearning and a passion for love that was inconceivable.

Life works in mysterious ways. So, on a warm November morning, I woke up from my sleep feeling a pleasantness I had not felt for weeks. I was on the mend.

I started to feel alive and hopeful. I engaged in exercise and healthy eating. Going to work kept me occupied, but just when you think you have it all together, life has a habit of knocking your socks off.

I developed Bursitis in my thigh from over-exerting myself. I had no option but to to see a physiotherapist. While at the physio, one very ordinary day, out of the blue I came across a long-lost friend who was also seeing the physio for some ailments. We became friends once again from the word go. I didn't look back. We picked up where we left off and she introduced me to her friends. Suddenly my loneliness subsided.

From the very beginning of meeting her friends, I felt welcomed by them. They were a bunch of fun-loving individuals, party animals. I was part of all the parties happening. I enjoyed planning and organising these fun parties with them. Little did I know the toll it would have on me further down the track. It was all unhealthy food we consumed. The sort that is quick and easy to prepare, nearly always accompanied by alcohol. I have always been health conscious, but because it was so much fun, I threw care to the wind.

The thought of facing life alone was not what I wanted, nor needed back then. Like the saying goes "if it makes you happy, go for it" and that I did. I engaged in their activities, which like I said earlier, were usually based around food and drink.

I became the designated party organiser, helping run dinner parties, Christmas parties, birthday parties and barbecues, all food-related activities.

There were six of us, so there were birthday parties all year round.

I stopped exercising and I indulged in the unhealthy foods we were consuming, and gained 10 kilos in weight in just eight months.

This was my lifestyle for two whole years. I figured it could be doing me harm, but the new found freedom and independence kept me engaged in the whole merry-go-round lifestyle. Consuming large amounts of unhealthy foods eventually took a toll on my body and mind. The worst thing of all was my sedentary lifestyle.

Unexpectedly, I received a call that took me by surprise. It was my ex-partner. In a dream-like sense of being, I heard him say "Joanne, I can't live without you". It was a voice I knew well. The words I wanted to hear. The man I wanted and missed. For a few seconds, I had to digest his words but then I heard myself say "Yes, I want you back".

This time around, he was in my life, but we lived apart. I introduced him to my party animal group of friends and his to mine. For quite a while we were all a big, happy family.

Life has many knocks, and this time the knock was a warning. Rod, who was one of my favourite friends, was a smoker, and a big soft teddy bear with a heart of gold. He unfortunately had numerous health issues. He was also very overweight. The news of him collapsing and dying in hospital from a heart attack was a wake-up call for me.
I decided to ease off and not attend the parties I was invited to. I needed time to reflect on what I was doing to my whole being. Unfortunately, I had realised too late.

Shortly after Rod's incident, I developed the pain in my abdomen. The hospital visit was the turning point for me.

My journey, the decisions I had to make, my research and my dietitian guidelines opened my eyes up to new possibilities.

I was becoming a new me.

I had discovered a new way of living and eating, so that was the beginning of my journey to wellness. It was easy for me to stick to as well, as I was an open book. And in the process I found a fountain of health. By adapting to this way of living I turned back the clock and found a way to heal my ailment.

It is now three years since that early morning waking in pain. It has been a recovery, but it's not a cure. I will need to follow the guidelines, keep eating for health and exercising for life.

I really think it's a great way to be fit, healthy and enjoy life.

If you are unhealthy, I am sure you wish you weren't.

You can do it.

It's just mind over matter.

Don't wait to be sick, don't be a slave to your demons.

There is not a better time than now to change your lifestyle and live a quality life.

I don't miss what I gave up. The parties, the unhealthy food. When you really think clearly about it, I really didn't need to moderate too much.

I chose to give up fast food, red meat and eggs. Previously, the hens couldn't lay eggs quick enough for the amount of eggs I was consuming, with bacon of course and melted cheese on top.

It took me a long time to get used to drinking my coffee without sugar, or drink coffee at all for that matter, as I have always been a non coffee drinker.

Recently, I was asked to organise a party for a friend of a friend. It was really more of a convenience party, as he organised to have a BBQ but the weather was not suitable for it. So I organised the party at my place, and in the process I ate hamburgers and fatty sausages that day, and leftovers the morning after. Not to mention the rich birthday cake, along with numerous beers and wine.

24 hours after the party, I awoke with mild pain in my abdomen. I quickly applied the remedies that I have found to work (refer to Chapter 7). It would be my first time trying the new found remedies on myself.

It took several hours of discomfort, but to my astonishment, the remedies worked.

The discomfort didn't eventuate into excruciating pain. By late afternoon, I still had the discomfort, at which time I decided to take two painkillers. I went to bed two hours later and woke the next morning pain-free. I was able to exercise for 45 minutes that morning with my fitness trainer and took my pooch for a long walk.

I was so happy waking up and examining myself, and to my delight, finding I was pain and discomfort free.

3 - THE DECISION THAT I HAD TO FACE

The outcome of my unwellness, in the early hours of that cold August morning of 2019, changed a lot of things for me. I could not comprehend the drastic decision put to me by the medical practitioner to have my gallbladder removed.

Why was there just one option presented to me by the doctor in charge?

I believe the decision I made to keep my gallbladder, made me a stronger and more certain individual than I have ever been before. I can now say this had a positive outcome and was right for me.

I'm not going to say that it was easy to be put on the spot. It was a difficult decision to make. I had to think quickly and logically, and it made no sense to me to take out my gallbladder at the first sign of malfunctioning. Surely they could have explained that there was a second choice. But it wasn't explained to me. I had to think for myself, look for other options, and not look back.

The symptoms doctors look for that indicate gallbladder problems are the following:

1. pain in the abdomen
2. yellowing of the skin or eyes
3. fever
4. vomiting
5. nausea
6. sweating
7. bloating
8. flatulence
9. coated tongue

The only symptoms I experienced, besides a lot of excruciating pain in my abdomen, were flatulence and perhaps a coated tongue.

After so many hours in hospital, and having had morphine administered for pain relief, the pain had not eased. But I had relaxed, and I was alert.

It was only after the stone miraculously passed that the pain subsided. Even after the stone had passed, I was still feeling quite tender under my ribs. If the stone in my bile duct had failed to pass on its own, I would have been taken to the theatre, where I would not have had any option but to have my gallbladder removed.

So I was lucky, and I was feeling pain-free to the degree that I was able to walk home from the hospital as it was only half an hour away.

I had suffered severe abdominal pain before without knowing its cause. Several years previously, I had been rushed to hospital and tests had been done. I believed at the time it was a psychosomatic pain I was suffering from. This was after the suicide of my first partner and the trauma and emotional pain I suffered.

As it turned out, after having more tests done, I was diagnosed with Helicobacter Pylori. I was also diagnosed as being lactose and fructose intolerant, at which point I decided to see a dietitian. I started to learn about gut health as it related to me.

Helicobacter Pylori is a very common bacterial infection, which raises the risk of stomach ulcers and stomach cancer. It is important not to have an overabundance of bacteria in your digestive system because it creates chronic inflammation, which can eventually lead to serious disease.

Infection in the stomach with the bacteria Helicobacter Pylori raises the risk of Cholecystitis - inflammation of the gallbladder. The presence of this bacteria also seems to be associated with cancer of the gallbladder or biliary tract.
Parasites and pathogenic organisms are attracted to a sick and dysfunctional digestive tract. You need to make your digestive system healthy and inhospitable to harmful bugs. There are excellent herbal products designed specifically to eradicate harmful microbes from the digestive system. Therefore, the most effective way to eradicate Helicobacter Pylori is to improve the health and function of your digestive system.

Failing that, Helicobacter Pylori can be treated by administering a dose or two of antibiotics. Since treating this, I have had no recurrence.

As I researched the gallbladder, I discovered that Helicobacter Pylori and the gallbladder are related. At the time, when I was admitted to hospital for abdominal pain, I did not know what I know now. I now understand why the doctor at the hospital told me that my gallbladder had to go and that it was an easy procedure.

He didn't suggest any other options, except to get rid of my gallbladder. The reason for this is that in many cases, medical students are taught very little about nutrition and lifestyle.

These have tremendous benefits for your general health and well-being.

Medical students will usually study body sciences such as anatomy, biochemistry, pathology and pharmacology. They also learn the basics of interviewing, examining, and treating a patient. However, the area of nutrition and lifestyle can sometimes be overlooked in their formal education. It has been reported that 80% of patients had conditions linked to lifestyle and diet.

For this reason, I decided to go to my doctor to get a referral to see a dietitian. To this day, I am happy that I decided to take the longer road, rather than the quick fix of removing my gallbladder.

Without a gallbladder, there's no place for bile to collect. Instead, your liver releases bile straight into the small intestine. This allows you to still digest most foods.

However, large amounts of fatty, greasy, or high-fibre foods become harder to digest. This can result in symptoms like loose stools or diarrhea, cramping, excess gas, and bloating.

Whether you keep your gallbladder or not, it will not alter your life span, but your diet and lifestyle will need to change.

4 – LOVING YOUR GALLBLADDER

A lot of things contribute to a lack of wellness. A gallstone doesn't just appear. It builds up over time.

Gallstones form when bile that is stored in the gallbladder hardens into stone-like material. Too much cholesterol, bile salts or bilirubin (bile pigment) can cause gallstones. When gallstones are present in the gallbladder itself, it is called cholelithiasis.

If stones are small enough, they may exit the gallbladder and pass through the bile ducts, into the intestine, where they are then excreted in your stool. When gallstones become stuck in the bile ducts, they can cause pain, obstruction and infection.

About 80% of people who have gallstones have "silent gallstones". This means they can experience no pain or symptoms their whole life. Bile aids in digestion, absorption, excretion, hormone metabolism and other functions.

Bile juice is a digestive fluid produced by the liver. It is stored and concentrated in the gallbladder. Its main function is to convert fats in food into fatty acids which are then absorbed in the gut.

Digestive System Diagram

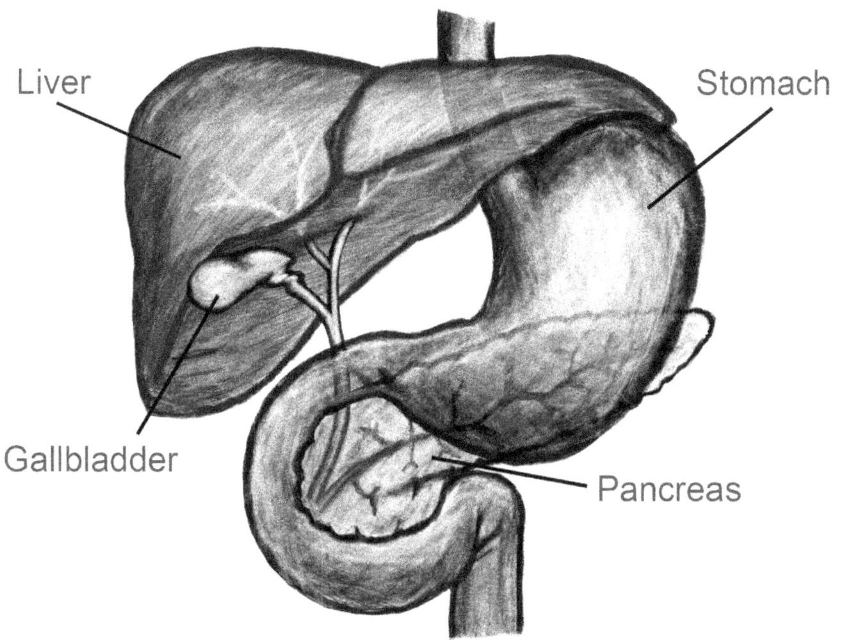

The gallbladder is a part of the digestive system. It is a small, pear-shaped organ located under your liver that stores and releases bile.

Bile is a fluid your liver produces that helps break down and digest fats in the foods you eat. It is made up of mainly cholesterol.

Before you start eating, your gallbladder is full of bile. When you start eating, your gallbladder receives signals to contract and squeeze the stored bile through the biliary tract.

The bile eventually finds its way to the largest bile duct, the common bile duct. Bile passes through the common bile duct into the duodenum, which is the first part of your small intestine, where it mixes with food waiting to be digested.

After you eat, your gallbladder is empty and resembles a deflated balloon waiting to be filled up again.

Several conditions can cause problems in your gallbladder, these include gallstones (cholelithiasis), inflammation of the gallbladder and biliary dysfunction (dyskinesia).

The function of the liver

The liver has various functions within the body, the main one being DETOXIFICATION. The liver helps to purify the blood by removing toxins such as alcohol and drugs from the body. It also helps regulate hormone levels. Hormones regulate everything from sleep to mood, metabolism, reproduction and immunity.

The liver works to DIGEST all food. Fats are digested by the bile in the stomach, which is a product secreted by your hepatic (liver) cells and transported to the gallbladder. Carbohydrates and proteins are broken down so that these nutrients can eventually be converted to energy for use within the body. Running alongside the liver, the pancreas is working to produce enzymes to assist in food break down.

The liver is the organ that makes bile. The bile goes into the gallbladder. An overloaded liver that produces unhealthy bile is the fundamental cause of gallstones. Exercise and diet allows the gallbladder to empty the bile sent from the liver.

The liver is also responsible for your IMMUNITY. It helps to get rid of bacteria, parasites and fungi.

Following are some ways to help your liver function at its best.

1.   Reduce your alcohol intake

Limiting your alcohol intake will improve your liver health. If you abstain from alcohol for one month, you can achieve peak liver function. If you must have a glass of wine, make it a glass of dry red wine as red wine contains antioxidants.

When I was focused on my healing, I made sure to keep my fluids up and would re-hydrate with water, fresh squeezed juices, teas and coffees.

2. Limit the amount of processed foots

Fats found in fatty processed meats like salami, ham, sausages and bacon, and deep fried foods like potato chips, are particularly bad for your gallbladder because they contain a lot of bad cholesterol.
If you must have chips, go for the frozen low cholesterol ones found in your supermarket and bake them in the oven. You could also make your own chips or wedges very easily (see recipe included) which will save in your pocket and in your gallbladder.

Cut out fast foods and only eat out occasionally. Biscuits, cakes and pastries have a high quantity of saturated fats, so it's best avoiding them altogether or find healthy alternatives in vegan recipes and make your own.

3. Increase your Omega-6 polyunsaturated fat

This will aid in reducing liver inflammation. Start working into your diet nuts, seeds (particularly flax seed) and good oils such as extra virgin olive oil.

4. Be smart with your selection of fruits

Eating certain fruits fresh, instead of processed, helps with absorbing the good acids and properties in their skins. These include blueberries, pomegranate and grapes, as these can help to regenerate liver cells. Also include in your diet, bitter fruits such as lemon and lime for their acidic properties.

After following this for a good month your liver should start to improve all its functions.

A note on weight

People who are overweight, especially women, are more likely to develop gallstones. This is because people who are overweight may have more cholesterol in their bile.

People who are overweight may also have a gallbladder that doesn't work as well.

Losing weight too quickly may raise your chances of forming gallstones as well. But slowly losing weight may help you prevent them.

In case of gallbladder surgery

If a person has too many gallbladder attacks, it's a sign that they may need to have their gallbladder removed.

Gallbladder surgery is not as intense as it sounds as it is only keyhole surgery and will leave no scars. If you have your gallbladder removed it is going to change the way you need to eat.

You can live without your gallbladder but it does help you digest fatty foods.

If you feel comfortable managing mild and infrequent gallstone attacks, and if your doctor thinks you aren't likely to have serious complications, it's okay not to have surgery. Most doctors recommend surgery if you have repeated attacks.

I started to make changes after my first gallbladder attack. Once was enough for me to have the wake up call I needed. Quick thinking, and the road I took, helped me keep my gallbladder.

5 - THE JOURNEY OF RECOVERY

This book is about all the steps that you need to take to bring yourself into a full, happy, healthy life. That is what your journey is about. These are some of the steps I took to bring myself into wellness, things which helped me on the long road of recovery.

My journey of recovery started from the word go. I bought a Pomeranian puppy that was to be my companion to help me get out and about to exercise. He is also the first four-legged flatmate I've ever had. It beats the two-legged homo sapiens. He asks no questions, he does not judge me, doesn't realise when I'm not wearing make-up and that I look a mess. He loves me unconditionally and I couldn't have made a better decision than to get him. He is the smartest dog, and I love him to bits.

I also invested in a treadmill, hoping to walk into health. I must admit, I do not use it every day but it does come in handy when I decide to walk. I walk at a fast pace. At first I could only manage five minutes of walking. I was so disappointed as at one time I could walk a whole hour, non-stop. But with some perseverance, I am happy to say I can now walk on the treadmill for half an hour continuously.

Occasionally, I go to the gym when I feel motivated. I also walk with a professional trainer for 45 minutes, fast walking once a week. At times, we will also box train, do stretch exercises and weight training.

I have also tried my hand at gardening. I am so lucky to have an art centre near where I live, which has garden plots of all different sizes and pricing. I hired a plot for $15 dollars a year. It has been a great time cultivating and growing organic vegetables, spending leisure time amongst nature, and seeing things grow. What a wonder! Best of all, I get to eat the fruits of my labour.

Music is so healing, and it so happens I love listening to great music, the sort that lifts your spirits. I prefer listening to music rather than sitting in front of the idiot box. I engage in writing poetry, and I am a member of a poetry group. I have also resumed keeping a personal diary, where I express my feelings and thoughts down on paper.

Mind and body connection

Good emotional health starts with being aware of your thoughts, feelings, and behaviours. Learning healthy ways to cope with stress and life's challenges is a part of life. Feeling good about yourself and having healthy relationships is very important.

Many things that happen in life can disrupt your emotional health. These can lead to strong feelings of sadness, stress or anxiety. Change - whether good to bad - can make life stressful.

These changes can include:
- A pandemic or global crisis
- Getting a job promotion or being laid from work
- Experiencing money problems
- Getting married or divorced
- Relationship problems
- Having or adopting a baby
- Moving into a new home

- Having a child leave or return home
- Suffering an illness or an injury
- Dealing with the death of a loved one
- A feeling of loneliness

Your body responds to the way you think, feel, and act. This is one type of "mind/ body connection". When you are stressed, anxious or upset, your body reacts physically. For example, you may develop high blood pressure or stomach ulcers after a particularly stressful event, such as the death of a loved one.

Path to improved emotional health

There are ways to improve your emotional health. Firstly, recognise your emotions and understand why you are having them. Sorting out the causes of sadness, stress and anxiety in your life can help you manage emotional health. Following are some other helpful tips.

Express your feelings in appropriate ways

If feelings of stress, sadness or anxiety are causing physical problems, keeping these feelings inside can make you feel worse. It's okay to let your loved ones know when something is bothering you.

However, keep in mind that your family and friends may not always be able to help you deal with your feelings appropriately. At these times, asking someone outside the situation for help can be useful.

Try asking your family doctor, a counsellor or religious advisor for support to help you improve your emotional health.

Live a balanced life
Focus on the things that you are grateful for in your life.

Try not to obsess about the problems at work, school or home that can lead to negative feelings. This doesn't mean you have to pretend to be happy when you feel stressed, anxious or upset. You may want to use a journal to keep track of things which make you feel happy or peaceful.

Research shows that having a positive outlook can improve your quality of life and give your health a boost. You may also need to find ways to let go of some things in your life that make you feel stressed and overwhelmed. Make time for things you enjoy.

Develop resilience

People with resilience are better at coping with stress in a healthy way. Resilience can be learned and strengthened with different strategies. These include having social support, keeping a positive view of yourself, accepting change, and keeping things in perspective. A counsellor or therapist can help you achieve this goal with cognitive behavioral therapy (CBT). Ask your doctor if this is a good idea for you.

Calm your mind

There are a variety of activities which can help you relax. Relaxation methods can include:
· meditation
· listening to music
· reading a book
· cooking
· art and creative expression
· yoga, tai chi and other forms of exercise

These and many other ways can help bring your emotion into balance.

Try new things and find what works for you. I have found guided imagery to be helpful for me, and there are free videos available on YouTube.

Take care of yourself

To have good emotional health, it's important to take care of your body by having a regular routine. This includes a routine of healthy meals, and exercise to relieve pent-up tension. Avoid overreacting and don't abuse drugs or alcohol. Using drugs or alcohol can cause other issues, such as family and health problems.

Things to consider

Poor emotional health can weaken your body's immune system. This makes you more likely to get colds and other infections during emotionally difficult times. Also, when you are feeling stressed, anxious, or upset, you may not take care of your health as well as you should. You may not feel like exercising, eating nutritious foods or taking medication that your doctor prescribes. You may abuse alcohol, tobacco or other drugs. These can all be signs of poor emotional health.

Why does the doctor need to know about your emotions?

You may not be used to talking to your doctor about your feelings or problems, but remember, they can't always tell that you're feeling stressed, anxious or upset just by looking at you. It's important to be honest with your doctor if you are having these feelings. First they will need to make sure that other health problems aren't causing your physical symptoms. If your symptoms aren't caused by other health problems, then you and your doctor can address the emotional causes of your symptoms.

Your doctor may suggest ways to treat your physical symptoms while you work together to improve your emotional health.

If necessary, your GP can refer you on to other specialists for extra support.

Since I had made my decision to keep my gallbladder, I needed to prove to myself that what I already knew about nutrition was correct. My first step was to make an appointment with my GP and discuss my options. I was disappointed that my GP was in favour of removing my gallbladder. Nevertheless, I asked him to refer me to a dietitian, which he happily did.

I had gained a lot of weight over a short time, and weighed more than I ever had. At the dietitian appointment, I was asked the reason for me wanting help. I eagerly explained my gallbladder dilemma, the amount of unhealthy foods I had consumed over time, and that I had become overweight. I had seen this particular dietitian in the past for my ailment of Helicobacter Pylori, so I had faith in her knowledge and understanding of her area of expertise.

I really believe food is medicine.

Many people have never been to a dietitian, so don't fully understand their contribution to our health.

Dietitians work with people of all age groups, cultures, food preferences and food allergies.

Dietitians will listen to their clients and what their lifestyle is like, and what their version of balance is.

They aren't speaking to you like a drill sergeant. Instead, they are having a respectful conversation and allowing you to make your own decisions.

The benefit of having a dietitian is that they can build a plan based on your needs and dietary preferences.

One of the conversations I had with my dietitian was about doing a gallbladder cleanse. I had been contemplating doing this, but there is much misinformation out there, and my dietitian was able to research this. She told me that this diet was unproven and again, let me make my own decisions.

6 - THINGS TO DO FOR A HEALTHY GALLBLADDER

1. Exercise

Regular physical activity can reduce cholesterol levels and help prevent gallstones from forming. Though small, gallstones can cause serious inflammation, pain, and infection. They can grow as large as a golf ball, but this is rare.

Maintaining a healthy weight and engaging in physical activity can reduce gallbladder pain and decrease the amount of gallbladder pain attacks. Through exercise and regular movement, gallstones can pass through naturally.

Ideally, it is recommended generally that people undertake half an hour of brisk walking or exercise movement 5 to 6 days a week. The benefit of this daily exercise is that it helps your liver and gallbladder function properly.

Consult with your doctor before performing any strenuous activity. While exercise is helpful, some activities cause strain on your abdomen and may worsen your symptoms.

2. Dietary changes

Poor eating habits, and consuming foods high in sugars and fats, can contribute to gallbladder disease and gallstones. A diet with less fat and more fibre can prevent gallstones and improve your health.

Fried foods, and other foods or condiments that contain fat - even salad dressings - are more difficult to break down and can cause gallbladder pain. Increasing nutrient-rich food in your diet, such as vegetables and fruits, can improve gallbladder function and prevent complications.

Some foods you should consider incorporating into your diet are:
- dark, leafy greens
- nuts
- brown rice
- whole grains
- fish
- olive oil
- beans
- citrus fruits
- low fat dairy

You should aim to include the above foods in your diet every day to decrease the chances of getting more gallstones, and having gallbladder attacks.

3. Peppermint tea

Peppermint contains menthol, a soothing compound that promotes pain relief. It can be used to ease stomach pain, improve digestion, and help relieve nausea and gas.

4. Apple cider vinegar

Raw apple cider vinegar contains anti-inflammatory properties that could be useful in relieving gallbladder pain.

To treat gallbladder pain, dilute 2 tablespoons of apple cider vinegar in warm water. Sip this tonic until the pain subsides. In your regular diet, apple cider vinegar can also be added to cold water, other beverages like juice, and worked into food recipes.

It's important not to drink apple cider vinegar straight, as the acid can damage your teeth, may cause digestive issues and affect potassium levels.

5. Turmeric

Turmeric is a spice used to treat many health conditions. Turmeric contains curcumin, which is known for its anti-inflammatory and healing benefits.

Turmeric stimulates the gallbladder to produce bile and helps the gallbladder empty itself. Incorporating turmeric into the diet can also reduce inflammation and gallbladder pain.

Turmeric can be made into a tea to drink daily for pain relief. The way I take it is by dissolving one teaspoon of turmeric in a glass of non-fat soy milk. Curcumin is also available as an oral supplement. Before taking any dietary supplements, discuss proper dosages and risks with your doctor.

6. Magnesium

Magnesium can be a helpful component for emptying your gallbladder. It can also ease gallbladder spasms and pain. Magnesium deficiency can increase the risk of gallstone formation. You can determine your magnesium levels by having a blood test. Magnesium is available at your pharmacy in powder form or as a capsule.

It is also found naturally in many foods particularly in certain fruits, vegetables and seeds. Discuss appropriate dosage with your doctor.

7. Water

Drinking water flushes away toxins from your body and empties your gallbladder. I cannot overemphasise how important water is for your wellbeing.

8. Dandelion root tea

Dandelion is a natural remedy which has been used historically to treat gallbladder problems, liver and bile duct issues. Its bitter roots may stimulate bile production in the liver which in turn helps the gallbladder function properly.

The polysaccharides in dandelion are known to reduce stress on the liver and support its ability to produce bile. Dandelion is an unusually nutritious food. Its leaves contain substantial levels of vitamins A, C, D and B complex as well as iron, magnesium, zinc, potassium, manganese, copper, choline, calcium, boron, and silicon.

You can purchase dandelion tea from your local supermarket. Do not take dandelion without medical advice, as it can interfere with certain medications.

You can drink dandelion tea like you would coffee. Some people substitute dandelion for coffee. The best and most potent way of drinking dandelion tea is by steeping a tea bag in boiling water, and drinking it black without sugar or milk, just like you would with herbal tea. If you don't like it black, you can drink it with milk and preferably no sugar.

9. Coffee

Moderate coffee intake - about 2-5 cups a day - is linked to a lower likelihood of type 2 diabetes, heart disease, liver and endometrial cancers, Parkinson's disease, and depression.

People who drink coffee have a 7 to 23 percent reduced risk of developing gallstones.

10. Get to a healthy weight

Being overweight or obese raises your chance of getting gallstones. That's because extra kilos can enlarge your gallbladder. This can cause your gallbladder to not work as well, which can in turn raise your cholesterol levels.

11. Load up with fruit and veggies

Fruits and greens are brimming with vitamins, including C and E. Both have shown to help protect against gallstones.

12. Cut back on fried foods

Your gallbladder has to work harder to help digest fatty foods. Fried foods are often high in saturated fat, which raises cholesterol in your blood. Eating a lot of greasy food can lead to gallstones.

13. Avoid crash diets

Crash diets can harm your heart and your gallbladder. That's because losing a lot of weight quickly keeps your gallbladder from emptying properly. To lose weight safely and steadily, aim to shed one to two kilos a week by eating sensibly and exercising.

14. Choose your alcohol wisely

Too much alcohol can harm the gallbladder, so limit yourself to no more than one drink a day for women and two drinks for men. Dry red wine has a much more positive effect than white wine as it contains antioxidants. Alcohol raises levels of HDL, or "good" cholesterol. It may have an effect on the cholesterol in bile. Go ahead, enjoy a glass of alcohol with dinner.

15. Watch your meat, butter and cheese

The fat in meat and dairy foods is saturated. This type of fat raises your bad cholesterol level, and in turn may make you more likely to get gallstones. Go for foods with non-saturated fats like those found in fish, chicken and vegetables instead.

16. Get moving

Physical activity burns calories, boosts mood, and protects your gallbladder. Women who exercise more lower their odds of having gallbladder disease by 25% compared to their couch potato peers. Aim for 30 minutes of workout five days a week. If you are just starting out, talk to your doctor about beginning with 5-10 minutes at a time. Every bit helps.

17. Go nuts

Nuts pack a lot of nutrition into a small size. They are high in fibre and healthy fat. They also have a lot of plant sterols, compounds that block your body from absorbing cholesterol. This may help protect against gallstones. Women who ate a handful of nuts five times a week were 25% less likely to need gallbladder surgery than those who ate them rarely. Snack on them, or sprinkle a few nuts on cereal, salads, and other dishes. Just watch the calories.

18. Lean towards vegetarian

You don't need to swear off meat for your gallbladder. But eating more meals with plant-based protein like beans and tofu may reduce the risk of gallbladder disease. That's because they're high in fibre and low in saturated fat. You might go vegetarian one day a week. Delicious meat-free meals include a tofu stir-fry, bean burritos, falafel wrap, and cheese and vegetable pizza.

19. Olive oil

This staple of the heart-healthy Mediterranean diet is also good for your gallbladder. It's a great source of unsaturated fat, which prompts your gallbladder to empty. When cooking, switch butter for olive oil. Other foods which contain healthy fats include salmon, nuts and avocados.

20. Heated compress

Applying heat can be soothing and relieve pain. For gallbladder health, a heated compress can calm spasms and relieve pressure from the bile build-up.

7 - REMEDIES AND
PAIN MANAGEMENT

The pain in my gallbladder started as an uncomfortable ache, and it eventuated into severe and agonising pain. At the time, I had no option and no understanding of the gallbladder and what triggers it to malfunction. I have explained in other chapters my story and my recovery and all the decisions I had to make.

I have also explained that by following my dietitian's guidelines, and by my own research, I have been able to live a normal life without any gallbladder dysfunction or pain since 2019. I have indulged in unhealthy foods without any issues. These would usually be bad for the gallbladder, but I have given myself a holiday from unhealthy eating for a while. Therefore, I can still integrate them as a treat. When you give yourself a break from eating these things constantly, you can enjoy them from time to time.

Sometimes I've gone off track and indulged myself. No matter how strict a person with their diet, there will always be temptation and everyone at some point drops the ball.

One evening, I hosted a BBQ party at my place, and I ate unhealthily.

There were fatty sausages, cheap hamburgers and birthday cake, washed down with beer and wine.

I threw care to the wind and I decided to enjoy the party and to indulge. I overate that night, and also ate leftovers for breakfast the following day. Being the host of the party meant that I was the one left with the fatty meats and the leftover cake. Who could resist?

In the middle of that night, I had gallbladder side effects of abdominal discomfort. I knew I needed to get up and stop it from getting worse. Since I have learned how to manage the discomfort, I knew I was going to be okay with the remedies that I have in place.

In this chapter, I will guide you through the things which have helped me stop discomfort from becoming great and unbearable pain.

I will explain to you how to recognise if you are experiencing gallbladder discomfort and how to deal with it.

Self Assessment

Lie down on your back on a bed, breathe in and hold it. At the same time, press with your fingers just under your right ribs. If you feel pain there, it is your gallbladder letting you know to act quickly before it gets any worse.

The following are the remedies that I believe worked for me, and hopefully for anyone else reading this book.

1. Peppermint tea

Peppermint contains menthol, a soothing compound that promotes pain relief. It can be used to ease stomach pain, improve digestion, and relieve nausea.

To ease gallbladder discomfort, you can drink peppermint tea.

Some think that drinking this tea regularly can reduce the amount of gallbladder pain attacks you may experience. Drink the tea black with no sugar. Wait 5 minutes to see how you're feeling. And if you still have the discomfort, keep drinking the tea regularly.

Peppermint tea relieves pain so it's good to drink plenty of it. It can take a full day to get rid of the discomfort and to keep it from becoming pain. When you are in this stage, it is important to be taking care of yourself. These other remedies will help too.

2. Apple cider vinegar

Raw apple cider vinegar contains anti-inflammatory properties that are useful in relieving gallbladder pain.

To treat gallbladder pain, dilute 2 tablespoons of apple cider vinegar with warm water. Or if you don't like it with water, do choose other alternative drinks like apple or orange juice. These are just some examples.

Sip this tonic until the pain subsides. It's important not to drink apple cider vinegar straight, as the acid damages your teeth. Drinking it straight causes digestive issues and affects potassium levels. Diluting apple cider vinegar before drinking it is vital.

3. Raw juice for gallbladder pain

Mix in a juicer the following ingredients:
5 fresh radishes
1 or 2 apples
1 fresh raw beetroot
1 fresh tomato
2 sticks of celery juice from
1 fresh lemon
2 carrots

This will make more than one glass of juice. You can drink some of the juice when it's blended and store the rest in the refrigerator for later use. Sitting up straight will allow digestion.

4. Magnesium

Magnesium can be a helpful component for gallbladder emptying. It can also ease gallbladder spasms and pain. Magnesium deficiency can increase the risk of gallstone formation.

To ease pain symptoms, mix a teaspoon of magnesium powder in warm water and drink every few hours. Magnesium is also available as an oral supplement. I have found oral supplements to be more effective and convenient. Discuss appropriate dosage with your doctor.

5. Water

Water keeps every system of the body functioning properly. Stay hydrated by drinking at least six to eight glasses of water per day. This helps keep bile production smooth. In addition, drinking water can also help flush out cholesterol from the body, which is one of the main factors that lead to the formation of gallstones.

Drinking water flushes away toxins from your body. Drinking water can eliminate or help relieve pain caused by a gallbladder attack. Many of these remedies involve drinking liquid, and so you can expect a few more bathroom visits during your day.

This is the self care that you show to relieve gallbladder discomfort. It is important to drink liquids sitting upright and keeping warm to give these remedies the best chance to be digested. And when it comes time to go to bed, don't go to bed with a full stomach.

6. Heated compress

Applying heat can be soothing and relieve pain. For gallbladder attack, a heated wheat bag compress can calm spasms and relieve pressure from bile buildup.

To relieve gallbladder pain, place the wheat bag in the microwave on high for two and a half to three minutes. You can also use a hot water bottle for the same effect, and apply it to the affected area for 10 to 15 minutes. Repeat this process until the pain goes away. It is very comforting.

Just be careful not to place the hot surface directly on your skin, as you could burn yourself.

7. Last but not least

It doesn't harm to try all the above when you feel discomfort. If a few hours have passed, and you still have tenderness under the ribs after examining yourself (as explained above), you can take two pain killers.

I can happily say I saved myself a trip to the emergency ward at the hospital by following the above steps.

Dealing with gallbladder discomfort in these ways can take up to a day to take full effect. The benefit of these above remedies is that it can reduce the likelihood of gallbladder discomfort developing into pain and attack.

8 - WHERE TO FROM HERE?

It's important to take care of both your body and mind. It will pay off in many ways including:
- Allowing you to take charge of your life and feel good about the choices you make
- Improving your overall physical and mental health
- Gaining energy and feeling fitter
- Gaining a positive outlook and finding more enjoyment in life
- Being a role model for your family and friends

Any lifestyle and dietary change is a work in progress. Whether you have a gallbladder problem or not, a healthy diet will improve all aspects of your physical and mental health.

So begin by setting small goals that are easy to add to your daily life and that you can control. Wellness and fitness include being aware and making healthy choices about diet, exercise and staying positive.

This is the most important investment you can make in your life. Strive for the best health you can have in all areas of your life by making mindful, healthy choices.

Path to improved health:
- Caring for your physical health through proper diet and nutrition whether meal preparation is for yourself or your family

- Focus on making smart, healthy meals that include greens, pulses and salads

Tips for success include:
- Make an effort to have more home-cooked meals. This can help encourage healthy eating. It also promotes more family time

- Keep healthy snacks on hand to help you make good choices. Have more fresh fruits, veggies and whole grains. Have fewer chips and sweets. Indulge in snacks like nuts, dark chocolate occasionally, fruit or healthy smoothies

- Teach yourself to eat when you're hungry, not when you're bored, sad or angry

- Breakfast helps jump start the day. It provides fuel for an active lifestyle and gives you the energy to think faster and more clearly. The best choice is porridge with berries and seeds

- Balance what you eat to meet your need for nutrition and enjoyment

- Focus on feeling comfortable instead of being full after you eat. Use moderation when choosing less nutritious foods. Eat slowly and have small meals

- A food and activity journal can help you understand your eating patterns. Also it can help you make simple, healthy changes. Ask your dietitian how to get started

- Limit screen time (TV, computer, video games). Consider other options like reading, board games or a family game of backyard cricket

- Choose to do activities you enjoy. Many people prefer walking. You can walk outdoors, at home on a treadmill, alone or with friends and family. Some exercise can be enjoyed while listening to music or audio books

- Try different activities like tennis, swimming, dancing, singing, cycling, team sports or yoga

- Schedule time to be active just as you would for any other important appointment

- Set short-term goals and plan rewards for yourself along the way

- Understand that life will sometimes get in the way of your plans. Stay flexible and get back on track right away

- Limit your exposure to friends who are not a positive influence in your life

- Get away from the office, school, or everyday life with day trips, weekends away or longer vacations

- Read an inspirational book

- Volunteer. Helping others can improve your emotional outlook

- Have a positive attitude. Tell yourself how great it feels to lead a healthy lifestyle

Things to consider

Don't let stress get you down. We all feel stressed at times. How you react to stress will determine it's affect on you. Take steps to prevent stress when you can and manage it when you can't.

Take care of you. It is important to be mindful of the choices you make for your personal health and well-being. Nothing is more important than taking care of you. Set aside time every day for yourself. Be active. Enjoy hobbies. Share time with your family and friends.

Personality traits like optimism and pessimism can affect many areas of your health and well-being. The positive thinking that typically comes with optimism is the key part of effective stress management.

A positive attitude can boost your energy, heighten your inner strength, inspire others and garner the fortitude to meet difficult challenges head on. Positive thinking can increase your lifespan, decrease depression, reduce levels of distress, offer better psychological and physical well-being and enable you to cope better during hardship and times of stress. Effective stress management is associated with many health benefits.

These are just some ideas about how you can make a difference to your health and well-being.

It takes a lot of courage to take the longer road and see yourself emerge like a butterfly from its cocoon. It feels great to realise that you have made the right choices. You may be in doubt at first but in time you will see the benefits.

I adopted the longer road, a road that led me into good habits, a life long journey, and a better way to live and heal. I began my journey in 2019 and I don't regret any decisions I made about my health. I am a stronger person for it today.

Even when I went against the doctor's suggestion, I admit I was in doubt but I trusted my intuition.

How are you loving your body? What steps are you taking to live a happy, healthy life?

You my readers may be facing a health issue. I have written this memoir for you. The contents of this book come from a lot of research but I am not a medical practitioner.

This book is my story about my journey from an unhealthy diet and lifestyle to a better me. I made a lot of changes along the road, things I would not have considered important back then. Everyone is different, every ailment is different. Not all gallbladders can be saved but all lives can be improved.

I hope by writing this memoir I have made you think outside the square. It's up to you, your gut feeling, your intuition, your courage. My aim in writing this memoir is to bring awareness and to hopefully inspire my readers.

I wish you all a full, happy and healthy life.

RECOMMENDED RECIPES

Breakfast

Ingredients
35g or ¼ cup rolled oats
¾ cup water or soy milk
Fruit of your choice eg banana, blueberries, strawberries
Chia seeds
1 tbspn honey Cinnamon

Method
In a small saucepan combine oats and water or milk.
Bring to the boil and stir for 3-4 minutes until desired
consistency is reached.
Pour into bowl.
Add honey and top with your favourite fruits and chia seeds.
Sprinkle over cinnamon to your liking and serve.

Orange, Avocado and Yoghurt Whip

Ingredients
1 avocado chopped coarsely
Juice of 2 oranges
1 dessertspoon of honey
Pinch of cinnamon
2 dessertspoons non-fat Greek yoghurt

Method
Blend all ingredients and enjoy.

Honey and Yoghurt Flip

Ingredients
1 cup non-fat Greek yoghurt
2 tbspns honey
1 tbspn toasted mixed seeds such as pumpkin, sesame and sunflower
Ground cinnamon

Method
Place the yoghurt, honey and half the seeds in a blender and blend briefly.
Pour into glass and top with remaining seeds.
Sprinkle with cinnamon and serve.

Note: This drink is great for gut health because of the yoghurt, honey and seeds. You could also add apple or banana as alternatives.

Carrot and Celery Juice

Ingredients
6 sticks celery trimmed
4 carrots trimmed

Method
Feed the celery and carrot through a juicer and serve.

Raw Juice

Ingredients
Mix the following ingredients in the juicer:
5 fresh radishes
1 or 2 apples
1 fresh raw beetroot cut in quarters
1 fresh tomato
2 sticks of celery cut to suit your juicer
Knob of ginger to your liking
Juice of 1 fresh lemon
2 carrots cut to suit

This recipe is good for gallbladder pain and your overall health.

Lunch Wraps

Ingredients
Lebanese or other flat bread
1 large ripe avocado
4 boiled eggs
50g baby spinach
2 tomatoes sliced
2 tbspns low-fat mayonnaise

Method
Mash eggs in a small bowl with a fork.
Add the mayonnaise.
Put aside.
Lay the Lebanese bread out on a clean surface.
Divide the avocado among the 4 pieces of bread and spread
evenly. Spoon egg and mayonnaise mixture evenly on top of the
avocado.
Top with tomato slices and baby spinach.
Roll up, and for an even more delicious wrap you can place it in
your sandwich maker for a few minutes to heat through.
The outside should be crispy.

Lunchtime tuna salad

Ingredients
 6 baby potatoes
1 red capsicum chopped
2 medium tomatoes quartered
1 lebanese cucumber halved and sliced
100g kalamata olives
2 hard boiled eggs quartered
½ cup basil leaves
2 x 200g cans tuna in brine
1 lemon or lime
1 tbspn olive oil
1 tbspn red wine vinegar
2 cloves garlic crushed
Handful of italian parsley chopped finely

Method
Cook baby potatoes in pot of boiling water until just tender.
Allow to cook then cut into quarters.
Put the potatoes, capsicum, tomato, cucumber, olives, eggs and
basil leaves in a large bowl.
Drain the tuna, remove from can and break up with a fork.
Add to other ingredients and gently combine.

Dressing
Combine lemon or lime, olive oil, red wine vinegar, parsley and
garlic in a jar.
Shake well.
Drizzle over salad.

Potato salad

Ingredients
1 whole potato
low fat natural yoghurt
wholegrain mustard
mint

Method
Cook a potato in the microwave.
Wash potato and prick the skin with a fork.
Place on a paper towel in microwave and cook 3 - 4 minutes on high, until soft.
You can dice up warm potato to make potato salad, mix with some low fat natural yogurt and wholegrain mustard, or mint.

Wedges

Ingredients
2 large white potatoes peeled (makes approximately 24 wedges)
Olive oil 2 cloves garlic crushed
Turmeric
Fresh herbs, ie basic, dill, rosemary

Method
Preheat oven to 200C.
Cut potatoes in half lengthways and then into wedges.
Place the wedges in a bowl or directly onto a baking tray.
Add olive oil, garlic, turmeric and herbs.
Combine all ingredients with your hands until wedges are well coated.
Place tray in oven and cook for approximately 30 minutes or cooked to your liking.

Note: You can use any herbs and spices you like. I like to use turmeric as it is a good anti-inflammatory.

Tabbouleh

This tabbouleh is really nice but you can buy it ready-made if
you don't have time to make it

Ingredients
1 cup burghul
4 medium tomatoes, chopped finely
2 Lebanese cucumbers, seeded and chopped finely
4 spring onions, sliced thinly
1 cup finely chopped fresh flat-leaf parsley
¼ cup lemon juice
1 clove garlic crushed

Method
Dry-fry burghul in a large frying pan over medium heat, stirring
for about 2 minutes or until browned lightly.
Transfer to a medium heatproof bowl.
Cover burghul with boiling water, stand about 10 minutes or
until burghul is tender.
Drain burghul, squeeze out excess liquid, return burghul to
bowl.
Stir tomato, cucumber, onion, parsley, juice and garlic into
burghul.

 Serve with chicken that has been lightly fried in olive oil and
sliced into 4 pieces.

Thai Chicken and Vegetable Stir Fry

Ingredients
Lemongrass or rind of ½ lemon
1cm/ ½ inch piece of fresh ginger
3 garlic cloves
2tbspn olive oil
275g lean chicken thinly sliced
½ red pepper sliced
½ green pepper sliced
4 spring onions chopped
2 medium carrots cut into matchsticks
150g green beans
25g peanuts lightly crushed
Oyster sauce to taste
Pinch of sugar Salt and black pepper
Coriander leaves to garnish
Chopped fresh chilli to your taste

Method
Thinly slice the lemongrass or lemon rind.
Peel and chop the ginger and garlic.
Heat oil in frying pan over a high heat.
Add the lemongrass or lemon rind, ginger, garlic and chilli, and stir fry for 30 seconds until golden.
Add the chicken and stir fry for 2 minutes then add all the vegetables and stir fry for 4-5 minutes until the chicken is cooked.
Finally, stir in the peanuts, oyster sauce, sugar and seasoning to taste. Stir fry until all the flavours are blended.
Serve at once sprinkled with the coriander leaves and accompanied by rice.

Note: You can use your favourite veggies instead of what is listed. I love to add broccoli and baby sweetcorn but it's up to you what you use.

Chicken Meatloaf

Ingredients
500g chicken mince
1 cup breadcrumbs
1 small onion chopped finely
1 carrot grated
½ cup shredded parmesan cheese
1 cup chopped fresh parsley
2 eggs
2 tbspns tomato paste
2 tbspns Worcestershire sauce
Barbecue sauce for basting

Method
Combine all ingredients in a bowl.
Pour into greased rectangular ovenproof dish.
Cook in 200°C oven for approximately 20 minutes or until nearly cooked.
Remove from oven and coat top of loaf with barbecue sauce.
Cook for a further 10 minutes.
Allow to cool for approximately 5 minutes and then slice.
Serve with your favourite vegetables or salad.

Tuna and Veggie Patties

Ingredients
1 medium carrot, grated
1 medium zucchini, grated
2 large free-range eggs
200g tinned tuna in brine, drained
40g parmesan cheese, grated
40g fresh breadcrumbs
2 spring onions, finely sliced
Salt Pepper 1 tbspn olive oil
1 lemon

Method
Squeeze out excess water from grated zucchini and carrot.
In a bowl, whisk the egg with a fork.
Add the tuna, parmesan and breadcrumbs.
Mix well.
Next stir in the carrot, zucchini and spring onion.
Season with salt and pepper.
Divide mixture into 4 patties.
Place a frying pan over low-medium heat and add the olive oil.
Place patties in frying pan and flatten with a spatula.
Cook for 2-4 minutes on each side or until patties have turned golden brown and are cooked through.
Eat as a burger, or with salad or veggies of your choice.

Apple Crumble

Ingredients
5 medium green cooking apples
3 tbspns water
3 tbspns castor sugar
3 cloves
1 cup wholemeal self-raising flour
2 tbspns butter
3 tbspns desiccated coconut
3 tbspns dark brown sugar

Method
Peel, core and slice apples.
Arrange in a pie dish with sugar, water and cloves.
Put aside.
Sift flour in a bowl.
Rub butter into flour until mixture is crumbly.
Add brown sugar and coconut.
Mix well.
Sprinkle over the apple mixture evenly.
Bake in 200°C oven until apples are tender.
Serve with custard or low-fat cream or ice cream.

Note: Other fruits such as rhubarb or apricots may be used
instead of apples.

Bran Muffins

Ingredients
500g wholemeal flour
50g unprocessed bran
1tspn baking powder
½ tspn salt
1 tbsp proactiv margarine
2 cups non-fat soy milk
1 cup honey
1 cup bicarbonate soda

Method
Combine flour, bran, baking powder and salt.
Rub in the margarine.
Heat the milk and honey together and add to the dry
ingredients with the bicarb soda.
Beat well.
Pour into greased muffin tins and bake in a moderate oven for
15-20 minutes or until cooked.

Date, Apple and Raisin Squares

Ingredients
4 apples diced
2 tbspn chopped walnuts
1 cup chopped dates
½ cup raisins
100g wholemeal self-raising flour
½ cup honey
½ tspn mixed spice
1 tbspn proactiv margarine

Method
Combine all ingredients mixing well.
Spread in well-oiled shallow baking tray.
Bake in a moderate oven for 30 minutes.
Cut into squares and serve warm.

EXAMPLE OF A MEAL PLAN

	SUNDAY	MONDAY	TUESDAY
Breakfast	Glass of Apple Juice with two tablespoons of Apple Cider Vinegar followed by bowl of porridge	Apple juice with two tablespoons of apple cider vinegar, followed by bowl of porridge	Apple juice with two tablespoons of apple cider vinegar, followed by bowl of porridge with strawberries.
Snack / Drink	Coffee with sugar and soy milk. Handful of nuts.	Coffee	Coffee
Lunch	Raw juice (as per recipe), tuna sandwich	Salad sandwich with avocado replacing butter or margarine	Sardines on toast.
Snack / Drink	Peppermint tea, one orange and handful of nuts	Peppermint tea, small bunch of grapes and an apple, fresh orange juice and handful of nuts	Peppermint Tea. One apple and handful of nuts.
Dinner	Bowl of homemade chicken and vegetable soup with chickpea	Thai chicken stir fry (as per recipe)	Grilled fresh salmon with squeeze of lemon served with greek salad (with lemon juice and a pinch of salt)
Dessert	Non-fat greek yoghurt with fresh fruit	No dessert	No dessert
Drink and Light Supper	Peppermint tea and veggie sticks with hommus	Leftover thai chicken stir fry. Peppermint and apple.	Veggie sticks with hommus, peppermint tea and one banana

WEDNESDAY	THURSDAY	FRIDAY	SATURDAY
Apple juice with two tablespoons of apple cider vinegar, followed by Weetbix with soy milk and honey	Apple juice with two tablespoons of apple cider vinegar, followed by homemade fresh fruit salad with non-fat greek yoghurt, sprinkled with nuts	Apple juice with two tablespoons of apple cider vinegar, followed by bowl of porridge with banana and honey. Coffee.	Apple juice with two tablespoons of apple cider vinegar, followed by muesli with sliced banana and soy milk. Coffee.
Coffee with handful of nuts	Coffee	Dandelion tea and handful of nuts.	Fresh squeezed juice (three oranges and one lemon). Peppermint tea.
Tinned salmon sandwich or on toast	Raw juice (as per recipe), lunch wrap (as per recipe), dandelion tea. One apple.	Leftover chicken meatloaf, with red kidney beans.	Tinned tuna (in brine) salad with avocado and chickpeas. Fresh fruit salad with non-fat greek yoghurt.
Dandelion tea. One apple.	Peppermint tea, non-fat greek yoghurt with grapes.	Peppermint tea, one apple and handful of nuts.	Coffee and handful of nuts
Vietnamese chicken noodle soup.	Chicken meatloaf (as per recipe) served with veggies.	Vegetable patty burger (as per recipe) topped with Greek salad.	Chicken with tabbouleh
No dessert	No dessert	No dessert	No dessert
Leftover Vietnamese chicken noodle soup. Peppermint tea and one apple	Leftover piece of meatloaf. Peppermint tea and one apple.	Leftover vegetable patty on toast. Peppermint tea and one apple.	Porridge. Raw juice (as per recipe). Glass of apple juice with apple cider vinegar. Dandelion tea.

ACKNOWLEDGEMENTS

This book came about after successfully completing a creative writing course. I want to give my gratitude to Donna Barrington from 'Respite Now', who was there with me encouraging and motivating me along the way. She has been a source of inspiration and moral support that kept me going to the end of my course, resulting in exceptional grades. Also for being involved in the process of writing this book.

I was also very lucky to have the support and the inspirational tutorial from my dietitian, Alex Salmon from 'healthAbility'. She is an excellent dietitian who was always there for me with her great knowledge of the value of nutrition for overall good health. Because of her support and encouragement, living well has become a way of life and routine for me now. She has been and always will be a great influence in my life.

I would also like to thank John Englezos from 'Sparrow Health' for being such a professional, fun-loving individual, and a great mentor. John helped me along the way to put this book together.

I am very proud of myself that this book is now in print which is something I would not have achieved if I did not have Donna and John's support behind me.

I would like to thank my psychologist, from 'Inspire Health and Medical' for all the emotional, motivational guidance and all the valuable therapy. They have been a source of inspiration. I look up to them with gratitude, for they are an exceptional psychologist and an amazing human being. I always left their office with a grateful and hopeful heart.

Thank you to Box Hill Hospital for all the good work they do. I appreciate all the care and support I have received from the incredible doctors, nurses, and staff over the years.

Thank you for all the encouragement of my dearest siblings and my dear friends.

Lastly to my four legged canine, Tigger, you make me happy.